MY HOSPITAL JOURNAL
A PRODUCT OF CANDIE PIE NATION

VISIT
CANDIEPIENATION.COM
for more products and helpful resources

HI THERE,

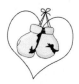

Thank you so much for supporting Candie Pie Nation! We're here to help in any way we can.

Hospital stays—especially prolonged ones—take a huge toll on our families, our loved ones and ourselves. Our routine, systems and sense of comfort are all suddenly replaced with uncharted territory.

It's like navigating a ship carrying the most important cargo in the world on stormy seas without a map. To say the least.

So, we're here to offer a helping hand. We're here to act as your map. We're here to make those waters a little less scary.

Use this journal to help you navigate. Use it to help you stay organized. Use it to help you remember. And, when all else fails, use it to bury your face in and scream. (We've been there, too.)

HERE'S TO YOU, CAPTAIN,
Diane & Candice (and all of your friends at Candie Pie Nation)

RESOURCES

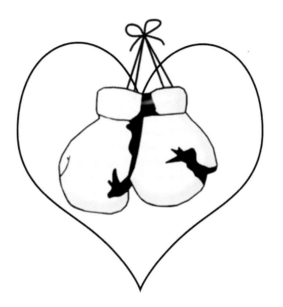

[Use this section to help you **navigate** your hospital stay.]

HELPFUL QUESTIONS
[to ask before a procedure or surgery]

Make sure you get your questions answered.
Be clear, concise and confident.
Doctors are busy. Pick your top 10 questions and ask how you can contact them if you have more.

- Is there anything else we can try or is this our only option?

- What will the doctor or surgeon be doing exactly?

- Do you have any pictures or diagrams to help me understand?

- How long is the procedure?

- Is there another way this can be done?

- Why do you prefer this way?

- What are the benefits? How long will they last?

- What are the risks or complications?

- Will there be more surgeries?

- What is your success rate?

- How often is this done?

- What needs to be done before to prepare? (Diet, medicine, etc.)

- Will there be a pre-op appointment? When and what will they do?

- Will there be any blood draws or other things that may scare my child immediately before the procedure?

- Can they have their favorite blanket or toy with them?

- Will they be awake?

- How long will they be under anesthesia?

- Will I be able to stay with my child or be with them until they are under?

- Where will I wait and who will update me?

- Who do I ask if I want an update?

- Where will they go after the procedure?

- When will I be able to see my child?

- What will they look like after, swollen, tubes, wires, monitors?

- How will they be feeling?

- What kind of medication will they need after?

- Will my child's health or condition make this more risky?

- How long is recovery? (Hospital and home) How long before my child can return to normal activities?

- Will there be another surgeon or doctor assisting?

- How do I explain this to my child?

- Do you know where I can get more helpful information about my child's condition or find a support group?

- How can I contact you if I have another question?

TAKE CARE OF YOURSELF
[stay positive & get mandatory rest.]

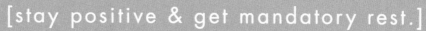

Remember: to fully be there for your **child**,
you need to **be there for yourself**.

_____

• Take breaks from the hospital. Ask if another family member or friend can sit with your child. See if a Child Life or hospital Volunteer can come to the room.

• Get some fresh air. Go for a walk or eat a meal outside.

• If you have other children, remember they need you too. Take time everyday to be with them. It can also help if they get a special trip to stay with family or friends.

• FaceTime or Skype with siblings or parents who can't be there. It's good for your child to hear and see their other family members in some way.

• Color, doodle or sketch. Some days, the only thing you can focus on is coloring. That's perfectly ok!

• Be crafty: Decorate your child's room. Make posters, hang up artwork your child or their siblings have made, post positive messages around the room, etc.

• Make a mailbox for visitors or nurses to write happy notes to your child. Read them daily. This can be very uplifting.

• Find local support groups who know what you're going through. Family and friends don't always understand and, sometimes, it's easiest to talk with an outside source.

• Smile and laugh, even if it's hard. Watch a funny movie, TV show or video on YouTube.

• Remember, people want to help you. Let them!

HOSPITAL BAG
[what to pack]

Always keep a bag **ready to go**.

If you're going to a doctor's appointment where you might possibly be sent to the hospital after, it's a **good idea** to bring the bag with you in the car **just in case**.

- Comfort Items: favorite toy and blanket

- Extra clothes, socks, underwear

- Things to stay occupied: books, activity books, coloring items, cards, small toys

- Pillow and nice blanket (if you know it will be a long stay)

- Snacks, water, hard candy, gum

- Personal hygiene items

- Medication list

- Phone charger

PEOPLE WANT TO HELP YOU
[learn to let them]

Accepting (and asking for) **help** is often one of the hardest things to do as a parent. But learning to **accept** help from others (especially during times like these when you most need it) can be **so beneficial** to you and your family.

Remember, the more help you get, the better off your child will be.

Don't be afraid to ask people for help with:

Laundry
Cleaning services
Grocery shopping
Paying a bill

Or, below are some gift basket ideas:

Family game night: Board games, cards, puzzles, candy

Coffee/Tea: Travel cups, coffee, tea bags, creamer, flavorings, sweetener

Movie night: Movie or iTunes gift card, popcorn, candy

Pasta dinner: Pasta, jar sauce, bread, salad kit.
(Put in a pasta pot instead of a gift basket.)

Mommy TLC: lotion, chapstick, sugar scrub, dry shampoo,
eye mask, ibuprofen, magazines, lavender spray

Daddy TLC: snacks, magazines, chapstick, lotion,
shaving supplies, small games

PEOPLE WANT TO HELP YOU
[learn to let them]

Below are even more ideas
of ways others can help:

Play date for siblings:
They also need a break and to feel special. Let others help you with this.

Gift cards:
groceries, gas, restaurants, iTunes, etc.

Meals:
Mealtrain.com is a great site to organize and schedule your meal deliveries. Sometimes, it can be a bit too much when people drop off food and want to stay for a visit. Don't be afraid to ask people to use meal delivery services.

At-Home Spa:
It is hard to get out to a spa, but every mom loves getting pampered. There are services where professionals will come to your house to do your hair and nails, and/or give a massage.

Car Maintenance:
It is so important to have a car to get to doctors' appointments and therapy. It is also hard to take a special-needs child with you to get an oil change or even just a car wash. Have someone take your car out for a wash, oil change and tune-up.

Cut out the below message and tape it to your hospital door to remind people your child can do far more with encouragement than they can with looks of pity or the words, "I'm sorry."

PUT ON YOUR GLOVES
AND GET IN MY CORNER

Please join me in staying **positive** and **strong**. Do not give me looks of pity or of sorrow. I am strong. **Stronger than you can imagine**. I am still here and **I am fighting**. I may get knocked down, but I have not given up. A trainer does not say to his fighter, "I'm sorry." A trainer doesn't feel pity for his fighter. A trainer understands a fighter's job is to fight. He cheers his fighter on. He has faith his fighter will win.

PLEASE HELP **CHEER ME ON**.
I WILL **WIN** THIS FIGHT.

THANK YOU FOR BEING IN MY CORNER.

HOSPITAL INFO
[writing things down helps.]

On (date)_____,

my child, (name)_____,

checked into (hospital name)_____

for (surgery or procedure)_____.

Our doctor is (name)_____.

Others helping me include (names):_____

_____

_____.

JOURNAL

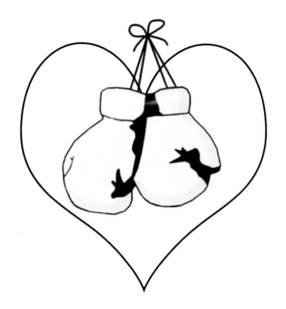

[Use this section to help you **document** your hospital stay.]

DATE:

My **positive** for today is:_____

Doctor:_____

Nurse:_____

Respiratory therapist:_____

Charge nurse:_____

How things look or feel today:_____

_____

I feel **good** about:_____

I'm concerned about:_____

I need to ask about:_____

I need to work on:_____

Specialist who visited today was:_____

They said:_____

Therapy I had today was:_____

Therapy Notes:_____

Test or procedure I had today:_____

I will get results:_____

DATE:

Today's Notes: _____

_____

_____

_____

_____

_____

_____

_____

_____

_____

_____

_____

_____

DATE:

My **positive** for today is:_____

Doctor:_____

Nurse:_____

Respiratory therapist:_____

Charge nurse:_____

How things look or feel today:_____

_____

I feel **good** about:_____

I'm concerned about:_____

I need to ask about:_____

I need to work on:_____

Specialist who visited today was:_____

They said:_____

Therapy I had today was:_____

Therapy Notes:_____

Test or procedure I had today:_____

I will get results:_____

DATE:

Today's Notes:_____

_____

_____

_____

_____

_____

_____

_____

_____

_____

_____

_____

_____

_____

_____

_____

DATE:

My **positive** for today is:_____

Doctor:_____

Nurse:_____

Respiratory therapist:_____

Charge nurse:_____

How things look or feel today:_____

_____

I feel **good** about:_____

I'm concerned about:_____

I need to ask about:_____

I need to work on:_____

Specialist who visited today was:_____

They said:_____

Therapy I had today was:_____

Therapy Notes:_____

Test or procedure I had today:_____

I will get results:_____

DATE:

Today's Notes: _____

_____

_____

_____

_____

_____

_____

_____

_____

_____

_____

_____

_____

DATE:

My **positive** for today is:_____

Doctor:_____

Nurse:_____

Respiratory therapist:_____

Charge nurse:_____

How things look or feel today:_____

_____

I feel **good** about:_____

I'm concerned about:_____

I need to ask about:_____

I need to work on:_____

Specialist who visited today was:_____

They said:_____

Therapy I had today was:_____

Therapy Notes:_____

Test or procedure I had today:_____

I will get results:_____

DATE:

Today's Notes:_____

_____

_____

_____

_____

_____

_____

_____

_____

_____

_____

_____

_____

DATE:

My **positive** for today is:_____

Doctor:_____

Nurse:_____

Respiratory therapist:_____

Charge nurse:_____

How things look or feel today:_____

_____

I feel **good** about:_____

I'm concerned about:_____

I need to ask about:_____

I need to work on:_____

Specialist who visited today was:_____

They said:_____

Therapy I had today was:_____

Therapy Notes:_____

Test or procedure I had today:_____

I will get results:_____

DATE:

Today's Notes:_____

_____

_____

_____

_____

_____

_____

_____

_____

_____

_____

_____

_____

_____

DATE:

My **positive** for today is:_____

Doctor:_____

Nurse:_____

Respiratory therapist:_____

Charge nurse:_____

How things look or feel today:_____

_____

I feel **good** about:_____

I'm concerned about:_____

I need to ask about:_____

I need to work on:_____

Specialist who visited today was:_____

They said:_____

Therapy I had today was:_____

Therapy Notes:_____

Test or procedure I had today:_____

I will get results:_____

DATE:

Today's Notes:_____

_____

_____

_____

_____

_____

_____

_____

_____

_____

_____

_____

_____

_____

_____

DATE:

My **positive** for today is:_____

Doctor:_____

Nurse:_____

Respiratory therapist:_____

Charge nurse:_____

How things look or feel today:_____

_____

I feel **good** about:_____

I'm concerned about:_____

I need to ask about:_____

I need to work on:_____

Specialist who visited today was:_____

They said:_____

Therapy I had today was:_____

Therapy Notes:_____

Test or procedure I had today:_____

I will get results:_____

DATE:

Today's Notes:_____

_____

_____

_____

_____

_____

_____

_____

_____

_____

_____

_____

_____

_____

_____

DATE:

My **positive** for today is:_____

Doctor:_____

Nurse:_____

Respiratory therapist:_____

Charge nurse:_____

How things look or feel today:_____
_____

I feel **good** about:_____

I'm concerned about:_____

I need to ask about:_____

I need to work on:_____

Specialist who visited today was:_____

They said:_____

Therapy I had today was:_____

Therapy Notes:_____

Test or procedure I had today:_____

I will get results:_____

DATE:

Today's Notes:_____

_____

_____

_____

_____

_____

_____

_____

_____

_____

_____

_____

_____

_____

DATE:

My **positive** for today is:_____

Doctor:_____

Nurse:_____

Respiratory therapist:_____

Charge nurse:_____

How things look or feel today:_____

_____

I feel **good** about:_____

I'm concerned about:_____

I need to ask about:_____

I need to work on:_____

Specialist who visited today was:_____

They said:_____

Therapy I had today was:_____

Therapy Notes:_____

Test or procedure I had today:_____

I will get results:_____

DATE:

Today's Notes:_____

_____

_____

_____

_____

_____

_____

_____

_____

_____

_____

_____

_____

_____

DATE:

My **positive** for today is:_____

Doctor:_____

Nurse:_____

Respiratory therapist:_____

Charge nurse:_____

How things look or feel today:_____

_____

I feel **good** about:_____

I'm concerned about:_____

I need to ask about:_____

I need to work on:_____

Specialist who visited today was:_____

They said:_____

Therapy I had today was:_____

Therapy Notes:_____

Test or procedure I had today:_____

I will get results:_____

DATE:

Today's Notes:_____

_____

_____

_____

_____

_____

_____

_____

_____

_____

_____

_____

_____

_____

DATE:

My **positive** for today is:_____

Doctor:_____

Nurse:_____

Respiratory therapist:_____

Charge nurse:_____

How things look or feel today:_____

_____

I feel **good** about:_____

I'm concerned about:_____

I need to ask about:_____

I need to work on:_____

Specialist who visited today was:_____

They said:_____

Therapy I had today was:_____

Therapy Notes:_____

Test or procedure I had today:_____

I will get results:_____

DATE:

Today's Notes:_____

_____

_____

_____

_____

_____

_____

_____

_____

_____

_____

_____

_____

DATE:

My **positive** for today is:_____

Doctor:_____

Nurse:_____

Respiratory therapist:_____

Charge nurse:_____

How things look or feel today:_____

_____

I feel **good** about:_____

I'm concerned about:_____

I need to ask about:_____

I need to work on:_____

Specialist who visited today was:_____

They said:_____

Therapy I had today was:_____

Therapy Notes:_____

Test or procedure I had today:_____

I will get results:_____

DATE:

Today's Notes:_____

_____

_____

_____

_____

_____

_____

_____

_____

_____

_____

_____

_____

DATE:

My **positive** for today is:_____

Doctor:_____

Nurse:_____

Respiratory therapist:_____

Charge nurse:_____

How things look or feel today:_____

_____

I feel **good** about:_____

I'm concerned about:_____

I need to ask about:_____

I need to work on:_____

Specialist who visited today was:_____

They said:_____

Therapy I had today was:_____

Therapy Notes:_____

Test or procedure I had today:_____

I will get results:_____

DATE:

Today's Notes:_____

_____

_____

_____

_____

_____

_____

_____

_____

_____

_____

_____

_____

_____

_____

DATE:

My **positive** for today is:_____

Doctor:_____

Nurse:_____

Respiratory therapist:_____

Charge nurse:_____

How things look or feel today:_____

_____

I feel **good** about:_____

I'm concerned about:_____

I need to ask about:_____

I need to work on:_____

Specialist who visited today was:_____

They said:_____

Therapy I had today was:_____

Therapy Notes:_____

Test or procedure I had today:_____

I will get results:_____

DATE:

Today's Notes:_____

_____

_____

_____

_____

_____

_____

_____

_____

_____

_____

_____

_____

_____

_____

DATE:

My **positive** for today is:_____

Doctor:_____

Nurse:_____

Respiratory therapist:_____

Charge nurse:_____

How things look or feel today:_____

_____

I feel **good** about:_____

I'm concerned about:_____

I need to ask about:_____

I need to work on:_____

Specialist who visited today was:_____

They said:_____

Therapy I had today was:_____

Therapy Notes:_____

Test or procedure I had today:_____

I will get results:_____

DATE:

Today's Notes:_____

_____

_____

_____

_____

_____

_____

_____

_____

_____

_____

_____

_____

_____

DATE:

My **positive** for today is:_____

Doctor:_____

Nurse:_____

Respiratory therapist:_____

Charge nurse:_____

How things look or feel today:_____

_____

I feel **good** about:_____

I'm concerned about:_____

I need to ask about:_____

I need to work on:_____

Specialist who visited today was:_____

They said:_____

Therapy I had today was:_____

Therapy Notes:_____

Test or procedure I had today:_____

I will get results:_____

DATE:

Today's Notes:_____

_____

_____

_____

_____

_____

_____

_____

_____

_____

_____

_____

_____

_____

DATE:

My **positive** for today is:_____

Doctor:_____

Nurse:_____

Respiratory therapist:_____

Charge nurse:_____

How things look or feel today:_____

_____

I feel **good** about:_____

I'm concerned about:_____

I need to ask about:_____

I need to work on:_____

Specialist who visited today was:_____

They said:_____

Therapy I had today was:_____

Therapy Notes:_____

Test or procedure I had today:_____

I will get results:_____

DATE:

Today's Notes: _____

_____

_____

_____

_____

_____

_____

_____

_____

_____

_____

_____

_____

_____

DATE:

My **positive** for today is:_____

Doctor:_____

Nurse:_____

Respiratory therapist:_____

Charge nurse:_____

How things look or feel today:_____

_____

I feel **good** about:_____

I'm concerned about:_____

I need to ask about:_____

I need to work on:_____

Specialist who visited today was:_____

They said:_____

Therapy I had today was:_____

Therapy Notes:_____

Test or procedure I had today:_____

I will get results:_____

DATE:

Today's Notes:_____

_____

_____

_____

_____

_____

_____

_____

_____

_____

_____

_____

_____

_____

DATE:

My **positive** for today is:_____

Doctor:_____

Nurse:_____

Respiratory therapist:_____

Charge nurse:_____

How things look or feel today:_____

_____

I feel **good** about:_____

I'm concerned about:_____

I need to ask about:_____

I need to work on:_____

Specialist who visited today was:_____

They said:_____

Therapy I had today was:_____

Therapy Notes:_____

Test or procedure I had today:_____

I will get results:_____

DATE:

Today's Notes:_____

_____

_____

_____

_____

_____

_____

_____

_____

_____

_____

_____

_____

_____

_____

DATE:

My **positive** for today is:_____

Doctor:_____

Nurse:_____

Respiratory therapist:_____

Charge nurse:_____

How things look or feel today:_____

_____

I feel **good** about:_____

I'm concerned about:_____

I need to ask about:_____

I need to work on:_____

Specialist who visited today was:_____

They said:_____

Therapy I had today was:_____

Therapy Notes:_____

Test or procedure I had today:_____

I will get results:_____

DATE:

Today's Notes: _____

_____

_____

_____

_____

_____

_____

_____

_____

_____

_____

_____

_____

_____

_____

DATE:

My **positive** for today is:_____

Doctor:_____

Nurse:_____

Respiratory therapist:_____

Charge nurse:_____

How things look or feel today:_____

_____

I feel **good** about:_____

I'm concerned about:_____

I need to ask about:_____

I need to work on:_____

Specialist who visited today was:_____

They said:_____

Therapy I had today was:_____

Therapy Notes:_____

Test or procedure I had today:_____

I will get results:_____

DATE:

Today's Notes:_____

_____

_____

_____

_____

_____

_____

_____

_____

_____

_____

_____

_____

_____

DATE:

My **positive** for today is:_____

Doctor:_____

Nurse:_____

Respiratory therapist:_____

Charge nurse:_____

How things look or feel today:_____

_____

I feel **good** about:_____

I'm concerned about:_____

I need to ask about:_____

I need to work on:_____

Specialist who visited today was:_____

They said:_____

Therapy I had today was:_____

Therapy Notes:_____

Test or procedure I had today:_____

I will get results:_____

DATE:

Today's Notes:_____

_____

_____

_____

_____

_____

_____

_____

_____

_____

_____

_____

_____

_____

DATE:

My **positive** for today is:_____

Doctor:_____

Nurse:_____

Respiratory therapist:_____

Charge nurse:_____

How things look or feel today:_____

_____

I feel **good** about:_____

I'm concerned about:_____

I need to ask about:_____

I need to work on:_____

Specialist who visited today was:_____

They said:_____

Therapy I had today was:_____

Therapy Notes:_____

Test or procedure I had today:_____

I will get results:_____

DATE:

Today's Notes:_____

_____

_____

_____

_____

_____

_____

_____

_____

_____

_____

_____

_____

_____

_____

DATE:

My **positive** for today is:_____

Doctor:_____

Nurse:_____

Respiratory therapist:_____

Charge nurse:_____

How things look or feel today:_____

_____

I feel **good** about:_____

I'm concerned about:_____

I need to ask about:_____

I need to work on:_____

Specialist who visited today was:_____

They said:_____

Therapy I had today was:_____

Therapy Notes:_____

Test or procedure I had today:_____

I will get results:_____

DATE:

Today's Notes:_____

_____

_____

_____

_____

_____

_____

_____

_____

_____

_____

_____

_____

_____

_____

DATE:

My **positive** for today is:_____

Doctor:_____

Nurse:_____

Respiratory therapist:_____

Charge nurse:_____

How things look or feel today:_____

_____

I feel **good** about:_____

I'm concerned about:_____

I need to ask about:_____

I need to work on:_____

Specialist who visited today was:_____

They said:_____

Therapy I had today was:_____

Therapy Notes:_____

Test or procedure I had today:_____

I will get results:_____

DATE:

Today's Notes:_____

_____

_____

_____

_____

_____

_____

_____

_____

_____

_____

_____

_____

_____

DATE:

My **positive** for today is:_____

Doctor:_____

Nurse:_____

Respiratory therapist:_____

Charge nurse:_____

How things look or feel today:_____

_____

I feel **good** about:_____

I'm concerned about:_____

I need to ask about:_____

I need to work on:_____

Specialist who visited today was:_____

They said:_____

Therapy I had today was:_____

Therapy Notes:_____

Test or procedure I had today:_____

I will get results:_____

DATE:

Today's Notes:_____

_____

_____

_____

_____

_____

_____

_____

_____

_____

_____

_____

_____

_____

DATE:

My **positive** for today is:_____

Doctor:_____

Nurse:_____

Respiratory therapist:_____

Charge nurse:_____

How things look or feel today:_____

_____

I feel **good** about:_____

I'm concerned about:_____

I need to ask about:_____

I need to work on:_____

Specialist who visited today was:_____

They said:_____

Therapy I had today was:_____

Therapy Notes:_____

Test or procedure I had today:_____

I will get results:_____

DATE:

Today's Notes: _____

_____

_____

_____

_____

_____

_____

_____

_____

_____

_____

_____

_____

DATE:

My **positive** for today is:_____

Doctor:_____

Nurse:_____

Respiratory therapist:_____

Charge nurse:_____

How things look or feel today:_____

_____

I feel **good** about:_____

I'm concerned about:_____

I need to ask about:_____

I need to work on:_____

Specialist who visited today was:_____

They said:_____

Therapy I had today was:_____

Therapy Notes:_____

Test or procedure I had today:_____

I will get results:_____

DATE:

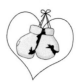

Today's Notes:_____

_____

_____

_____

_____

_____

_____

_____

_____

_____

_____

_____

_____

_____

Made in United States
Orlando, FL
06 September 2024